PATANJALI YOGA SÛTRAS

TO BE PRESENT IN YOGA

Graphic Design

Mattias Långström

Contact: oneofakindbooks@bhagwan.se

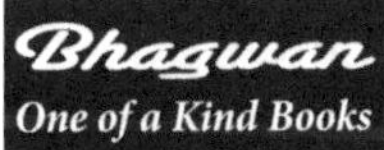

Patanjali Yoga Sûtras

TO BE PRESENT IN YOGA

Translation and comments
Jan Fahleman

✳✳✳

Copyright © Jan Fahleman

Contact: oneofakindbooks@bhagwan.se

Published by **BHAGWAN 2021**

No part of this publication may be reproduced or transmitted in any form, or by any means, electronic or mechanical, including photocopying, scanning, recording, or any information storage and retrieval sýstem, without express written permission from the publisher, except for the inclusion of brief quotations embodied in critical articles and reviews. This book is a work of fiction and a product of the author´s imagination.

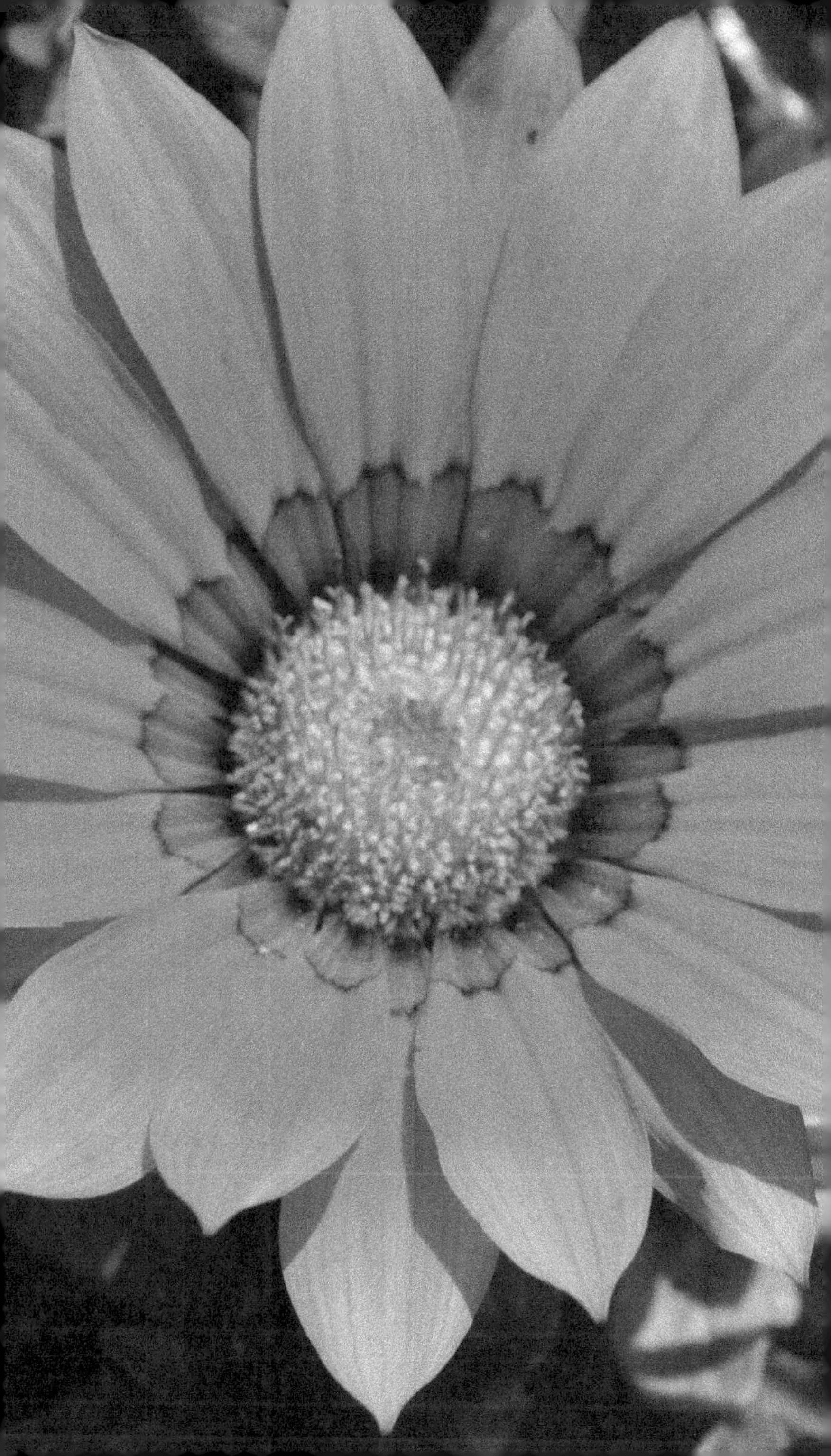

Introduction

Yoga Sutras by Patanjali has achieved the status of being one of the most important classical yoga texts and Patanjali's definition of yoga is also one of the most widespread. He was the first to methodically record the ancient and timeless knowledge of yoga in eight classical steps. With Patanjali, yoga was incorporated into the Hindu tradition as one of six philosophical paths and gained its distinct Indian character.

A good way to approach the knowledge is to read a few sutras at a time. They are logical in their structure and you will slowly understand more and more.

Patanjali's classic sutras are carefully interpreted by the Swedish author Jan Fahleman. He has practiced meditation and yoga asanas for many decades and applied some of Patanjali's sutras. He has studied Vedic literature and various spiritual masters since the 1970s.

Preface

Patañjali lived about 200 years B.C. in India. There is little historical information about him. He has often been called Maharishi Patañjali. In his work "Yoga Sutras" he explained and described yoga with 196 short sutras. These sutras can be seen as formulas or aphorisms of philosophical wisdom. They were originally not written down but were passed on orally from teacher to student.

The word Yoga can be derived from the Sanskrit word yuj which means union and refers to union with the divine. This compound is not an event that will happen in the future, it occurs in the present, but the individual must be aware of this relationship. Patañjali describes in his sutras how the obstacles to this awareness can be bridged. He gives instructions on eight paths for practical application. Patanjali's theoretical philosophy can be verified by experience through practical application.

Unfortunately, there are many of misconceptions when it comes to yoga. The prevailing view is that yoga is mostly different postures called asanas. Patanjali explains that Yoga asanas is but one of the eight paths that can lead to the state of Consciousness called yoga or Samādhi.

I have chosen to write simply and understandably, with expressions and terms that many spiritual teachers use today. My starting point was Patanjali's original text in Sanskrit, but in my comments also draw from my own personal experience of yoga. I have written comments where I experienced the need for a clarification and have tried to keep these comments as brief as possible.

Throughout, the Sanskrit and the transliterated texts are on the left page and the english translation is on the right side one.

Jan Fahleman
Stockholm 2021

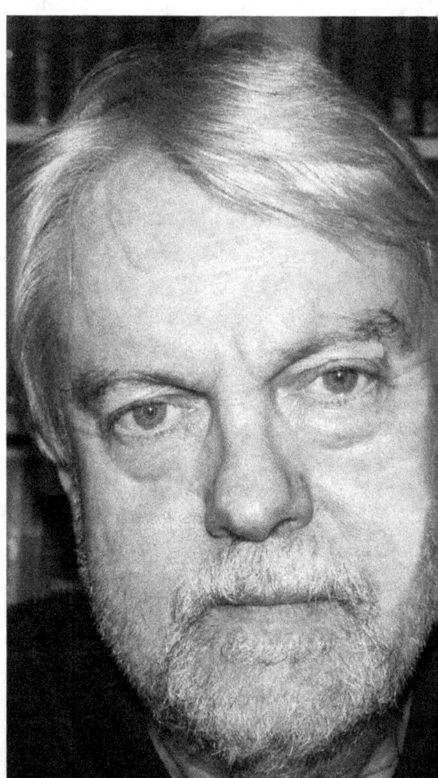

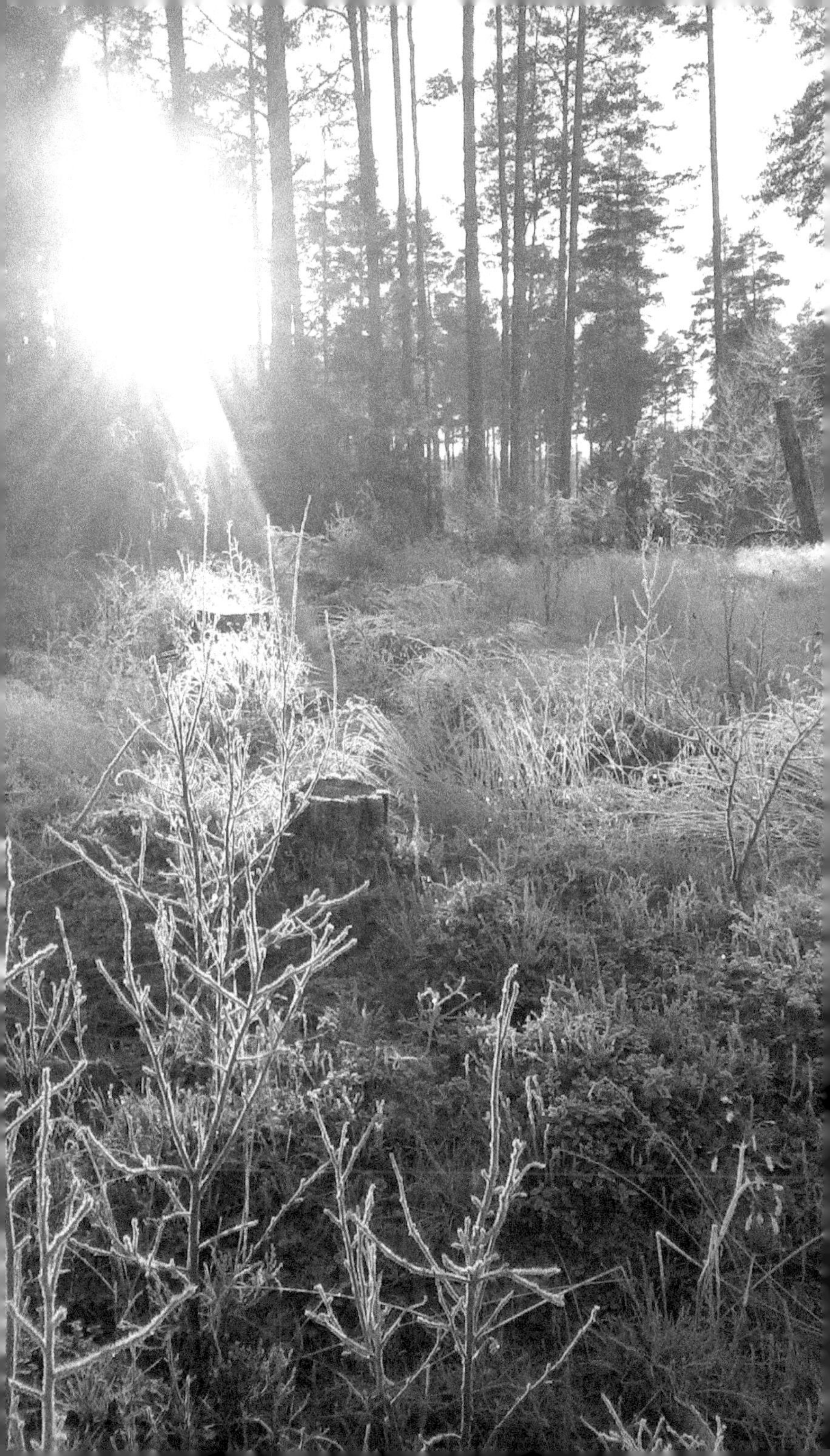

Chapter 1

SAMĀDHI PĀDA

About the state of awareness named

Samādhi

अथ योगानुशासनम्॥१॥

1. Atha yogānuśāsanam

योगश्चित्तवृत्तनिरोधः॥२॥

2. Yogaś citta vṛtti nirodhaḥ

तदा द्रष्टुः स्वरूपेऽवस्थानम्॥३॥

3. Tadā draṣṭuḥ svarūpe'vasthānam

वृत्तिसारूप्यमितरत्र॥४॥

4. Vṛtti sārūpyam itaratra

वृत्तयः पञ्चतय्यः क्लिष्टा अक्लिष्टाः॥५॥

5. Vṛttayaḥ pañcatayyaḥ kliṣṭā akliṣṭāḥ

1. Here begins the exposition of Yoga.

2. Yoga arises when awareness is no longer bound by the mind.

To be in the state of "Yoga", requires that the senses ie. thoughts, emotions and objects are not obstacles. The sense perceptions may continue to exist, but awareness is no longer bound by them in the state of yoga.

(Awareness is the individual focus and presence that provides experiences in the present).

3. Then the seer is aware of itself.

When the seer is aware of the Self, ie. is present in Consciousness, the true identity is revealed. The identity created by the mind is then seen as false, unreal and created out of ignorance.

(Consciousness is the absolute pure cosmic Consciousness that has many names: God, the Holy Spirit, the Spirit, Self, Being, Tao, or Brahman. Few words have so many prejudices and definitions as the word God. God is often referenced to a being in the outer life that one is separated from. Therefore Consciousness a better word in this context.)

4. Otherwise Consciousness is identified with the sensations.

Merely being aware of mental activity and sensory objects implies a limitation in experience of life. Obviously, it's good to be able to be present in the mind, but it may prevent the presence of Consciousness.

5. There are five different state of mind, some creates suffering while others do not.

In the relative changing life there is both happiness and suffering. As long as awareness is tied to the mind, both suffering and happiness will be experienced.

परमाणवपिर्ययवकिल्पनिद्रास्मृतयः॥६॥

6. Pramāṇa viparyaya vikalpa nidrā smṛtayaḥ

प्रत्यक्षानुमानागमाः प्रमाणानि॥७॥

7. Pratyakṣānumānāgamāḥ pramāṇāni

वपिर्ययो मथियाज्ञानमतद्रूपप्रतष्ठिम्॥८॥

8. Viparyayo mithyā-jñānam atad-rūpa pratiṣṭham

शब्दज्ञानानुपाती वस्तुशून्यो वकिल्पः॥९॥

9. Śabda-jñānānupātī vastu-śūnyo vikalpaḥ

अभावप्रत्ययालम्बना वृत्तिर्निद्रा॥१०॥

10. Abhā-vapratyayālambanā vṛttir nidrā

6. *They are; (pramana) valid knowledge (viparyaya) ignorance, (vikalpa) illusion (nidra) sleep and (smrti) memory.*

7. *Valid knowledge (pramana) is obtained by direct experience, by drawing conclusions and by external testimony.*

This knowledge is obtained through the sense organs and by the intellect, which draws conclusions and by information coming from the environment. This is relative knowledge which the mind handles.

8. *Ignorance (viparyaya) arises from misinterpretation of what is experienced.*

The mind often wants to interpret what is perceived to fit with the situation that the mind is experiencing. This experience is often related to the past but also to an anticipated future, but it's not always this interpretation is consistent with the reality of the present.

9. *Illusion (vikalpa) is to imagine something that does not exist.*

The mind can create and fantasize a mental reality that is an illusion. Problems can arise if these "castles in the air" are used as true reality. In the yoga literature one often uses an example with a rope taken for a snake to illustrate this. In the dark one is mistaken thinking that a rope is a snake which evokes fear. When the light is turned on, you see reality, ie. that the thing on the floor is a rope and that the snake is a mental illusion.

10. Sleep (nidrā) is the mental state characterized by the absence of awareness.

The dreamless sleep is characterized by non-mental activity.

अनुभूतवषियासम्परमोषः स्मृतिः॥११॥

11. Anubhūta-viṣayāsampramoṣaḥ smṛtiḥ

अभ्यासवैराग्याभ्यां तन्निरोधः॥१२॥

12. Abhyāsa-vairāgyābhyāṁ tan-nirodhaḥ

तत्र स्थितौ यत्नोऽभ्यासः॥१३॥

13. Tatra sthitau yatno'bhyāsah

स तु दीर्घकालनैरन्तर्यसत्कारासेवतो दृढभूमिः॥१४॥

14. Sa tu dīrgha-kāla-nairantarya-satkārāsevito
      dṛdha-bhūmih

दृष्टानुश्रवकिवषियवतृष्णस्य वशीकारसञ्ज्ञा
वैराग्यम्॥१५॥

15. Dṛṣṭānuśravika-viṣaya-vitṛṣnasya vaśīkāra-
      sañjñā vairāgyam

11. Memory (smrti) is the mental ability to become aware of past experiences.

Memory is a tool for the intellect that needs memory to be able to draw conclusions from previous experiences.

12. These sensory sensations can be mastered through practice and attitude.

To be bound to the mind means to be a victim in the relative existence. This does not mean that the mind will be destroyed. The mind with its senses is an excellent tool for navigating in the relative existence. Witnessing the mind by being consciously present in the Conscio-usness means that one can master the mind. Practicing this approach leads to liberation.

13. By practicing and exercising (abhyāsa) conditions for presence in consciousness arise.

Becoming aware of Consciousness can happen in different ways. One way to become aware is to practice different exercises.

14. Practicing regularly and with dedication for a long time, provides a solid foundation.

Practicing can mean being vigilant and present. It enables an awareness, which provides a stable foundation. The reason for vigilance is that the mind and senses constantly want all the attention, which can mean that the awareness of Consciousness is lost.

15. When independence (vairāgyā) prevails, awareness is no longer bound by the senses and can then be present in Consciousness. This is a state of self-sufficiency. There is then no need to seek sensual satisfaction.

When awareness can be present in Consciousness, freedom and self-sufficiency arise. There is then no need to search for pleasures, wealth and power. In this state of Consciousness, it is obvious that pleasures, possessions and positions of power do not provide real freedom and satisfaction.

तत्परं पुरुषख्यातेर्गुणवैतृष्ण्यम्॥१६॥

16. Tat paraṁ puruṣa-khyāter guṇavaitṛṣṇyam

वितर्कवचिारानन्दास्मितिरूपानुगमात्सम्प्रज्ञा
तः॥१७॥

17. Vitarka-vicārānandāsmitārūpānugamāt
samprajñātaḥ

वरिामप्रत्ययाभ्यासपूर्वः संस्कारशेषोऽन्यः॥१८॥

18. Virāma pratyayābhyāsa-pūrvaḥ
saṁskāra-śeṣo'nyaḥ

भवप्रत्ययो वदिेहप्रकृतिलियानाम्॥१९॥

19. Bhavapratyayo videhaprakṛtilayānām

16. By experiencing Purusa (Consciousness) a state of freedom arises when the attachment to the qualities of the relative changing existence (gunas) has ceased.

In this state of independence, the mind, ego, intellect and body continue to function, even they continue to function in a more harmonious and coordinated way, but they are no longer an obstacle to the presence of Consciousness. By experiencing Consciousness, which is free from all influence and the three gunas, the true identity is experienced, which witnesses the relative sensory sensations without being bound by them and the relatively changing existence, the three gunas. These qualities and energies are; tamas which is characterized as inertia, cruelty and low energy, rajas as activity, desire and active energy and sattva as goodness, truth and pure energy. It is always one of the three gunas that dominates the present in the relative existence.

17. Samprajñātah samādhi, is called the state of Consciousness that integrates insight and wisdom as well as happiness with the experience of Consciousness.

In this state of Consciousness, which is free from attachment, understanding and insights come as a matter of course. No intellectual processing is required and no external information, from e.g. literature or from a teacher. Happiness and peace arise spontaneously without any sensation being the cause.

18. In Asamprajñāta-samādhi there are no sensory sensations, but memories of past experiences remain.

The state of Consciousness Samādhi does not mean an extinction of individuality. Experiences and memories that make up the individual's life history and experience bank are still latent.

19. There are those called videhas and prakrtilayas who have innate abilities that enable them to be reconciled with nature without practice and explanation.

For some people, the insight and understanding of the relationship between the observer, the observed and the process of observing is so established and obvious that no explanations or exercises are needed to experience it.

शरद्धावीर्यस्मृतिसिमाधिप्रज्ञापूर्वक इतरेषाम्॥२०॥

20. Śraddhā-vīrya-smṛti-samādhi-prajñāpūrvaka
itareṣām

तीव्रसंवेगानामासन्नः॥२१॥

21. Tīvra-saṁvegānām āsannaḥ

मृदुमध्याधिमात्रत्वात्ततोऽपि विशेषः॥२२॥

22. Mṛdu-madhyādhimātratvāt tato 'pi viśeṣaḥ

ईश्वरप्ररणधिानाद्वा॥२३॥

23. Īśvara-praṇidhānād vā

क्लेशकर्मविपाकाशयैरपरामृष्टः पुरुषविशेष
ईश्वरः॥२४॥

24. Kleśakarmavipākāśayairaparāmṛṣṭaḥ
puruṣaviśeṣa īśvaraḥ

*20. Others use knowledge, trust and spiritual discipline
to establish the Asamprajñāta-samādhi level of consciousness.*

*Being focused and present is the basis for being aware
of the consciousness. Knowledge, trust and spiritual
discipline are tools that can be helpful.*

*21. He who is focused and has a strong desire soon
reaches the state of consciousness samādhi.*

*If the desire is strong and established on an active cons-
cious level, life will be focused on satisfying this desire as
soon as possible.*

*22. The degree of commitment to reach samādhi, varies
from small to moderate or intense.*

*At different times during a life cycle, the conditions can
vary when it comes to focusing on and devoting time to,
a commitment to reach Samādhi. Both the prevailing
life situation and the intensity of the desire to reach
samādhi affect the intensity of the yoga practice.*

*23. By surrendering to Īśvara (the consciousness of
God), realization can also take place.*

When awareness is present in Consciousness, Samādhi is a fact. This association is not bound to anything that will happen in the future as Consciousness is already present and has always existed. It is not something that needs to be created or developed but can be experienced here and now, but there must be a desire and a willingness to cooperate to surrender to God. This is called Bhakti Yoga.

24. Īśvara is not bound by karma and suffering.
Īśvara is a personal aspect of Purusa (Consciousness). But this divine personality is not affected like other personalities by karma. The meaning of karma is that actions create repercussions that affect the individual. Karma is a way of educating the individual through problems and suffering creating desires for a better life situation. Īśvara which is already perfect and self-sufficient does not need to be nurtured through karma.

तत्र निरतिशियं सर्वज्ञवीजम्॥२५॥

25. Tatra niratiśayaṁ sarvajñatva beejam

पूर्वेषामपि गुरुः कालेनानवच्छेदात्॥२६॥

26. Sa pūrveṣāmapi guruḥ kālenānavacchedāt

तस्य वाचकः प्रणवः॥२७॥

27. Tasya vācakaḥ praṇavaḥ

तज्जपस्तदर्थभावनम्॥२८॥

28. Tajjapas tad-artha-bhāvanam

ततः प्रत्यक्चेतनाधिगमोऽप्यन्तरायाभावश्च॥२९॥

29. Tataḥ pratyak-cetanādhigamo'py an-
       tarāyā-bhāvaś ca

*25. Īśvara, is the seed of the origin of everything, is
omniscient.*

*The God-consciousness has total knowledge, control and
presence both in the manifested relative existence and
the absolute being, the unmanifested existence.*
*26. The divine, independent of time, is the teacher of the
teachers of all ages.*

*The knowledge transmitted from the consciousness of
God is independent of time. It is independent of the
prevailing spirit of the times. This means that the same
knowledge is conveyed from the consciousness of God
regardless of the age that prevails. What may vary is the
susceptibility that may be different in different eras.*

*27. The divine manifests itself as pranavah in the form
of Āum (Om).*

*Āum or Om is a sound that has the quality and energy
of the divine and that permeates and vibrates throughout the whole of relative existence. It is a "divine music"
that one can pay attention to and use as a mantra in
meditation.*

*28. One should constantly repeat and pay attention to
Om.*

Focusing and keeping attention on the mantra Om, means that the mantra´s qualities and energy have prescence in the mind. There are then conditions for contact with Consciousness.

29. *In this way the obstacles can be removed and then the possibility arises that Consciousness can be experienced.*

The effects of being focused and present in Om can be both mental and physical healing. In this way, attention can go from problems and suffering to experiencing Consciousness as the real and true identity.

व्याधिस्त्यानसंशयप्रमादालस्याविरतिभिरा
न्तदर्शनालब्धभूमिकत्वानवस्थितत्वानि
चित्तविक्षेपास्तेऽन्तरायाः ॥३०॥

30. Vyādhi- styāna-saṁśaya-pramādālasyā-vira-
ti-bhrānti-darśanālabdhabhūmi-katvānavasthitat-
vāni citta-vikṣepās te 'ntarāyāḥ

दुःखदौर्मनस्याङ्गमेजयत्वश्वासप्रश्वासा
वक्षेपसहभुवः ॥३१॥

31. Duḥkha-daurmanasyāṅgamejayatva-śvāsa-
praśvāsā vikṣepa-sahabhuvaḥ

तत्प्रतिषिधार्थमेकतत्त्वाभ्यासः ॥३२॥

32. Tat-pratiṣedhārtham eka-tattvābhyāsaḥ

मैत्रीकरुणामुदितोपेक्षाणां
सुखदुःखपुण्यापुण्यविषियाणां
भावनातश्चित्तप्रसादनम् ॥३३॥

33. Maitrī-karuṇā-muditopekṣāṇāṁ sukha-duḥk-
ha-puṇyāpuṇya-viṣayāṇāṁ bhāvanātaś-cit-
ta-prasādanam

30. *Illness, lethargy, doubt, thoughtlessness, listlessness, delusion, difficulty in concentrating and instability are the factors that appear to be obstacles.*

The nine factors listed are characteristics of a awareness that is bound to the mind and lacks conscious anchoring in Consciousness. Since these factors are obstacles, they must be a way out of this mental prison.

31. *Suffering, anxiety, tremors in the body and irregular breathing may be the result of this state of Consciousness.*

This state of Consciousness eventually results in an overload in the nervous system, which then causes problems in various bodily functions and mental disorders. Today we usually call this condition "stress".

32. *Removing these obstacles requires focused and regular practice.*

Getting out of that mental prison may require a regular commitment of being focused and present in appropriate exercises, in order to thereby make the awareness change focus.

33. *When peace and quiet prevail, the reaction to the*

surroundings takes on these qualities; kindness and fellowship with the happy, compassion and love for the unhappy and suffering, neutrality and indifference to the wicked.

Evil can be dealt with in different ways; meeting evil with evil reinforces evil, meeting it with love can in some cases reduce evil, but in other situations evil can be strengthened by feeling threatened. Approaching evil with neutrality and indifference can mean that evil remains latent and inactive. To behave consciously present rooted in the Consciousness, adapted to the prevailing situation, is the best approach, to evil.

परच्छर्दनविधारणाभ्यां वा प्राणस्य॥३४॥

34. Pracchardana-vidhāraṇābhyāṁ vā prāṇasya

विषयवती वा प्रवृत्तिरुत्पन्ना मनसः
स्थतिनिबिन्धनी॥३५॥

35.Viṣayavatī vā pravṛttir utpannā manasaḥ st-
hiti-nibandhainī

विशोका वा ज्योतिष्मती॥३६॥

36. Viśokā vā jyotiṣmatī

वीतरागवषियं वा चत्तितम्॥३७॥

37. Vīta-rāga-viṣayaṁ vā cittam

स्वप्नननिद्राज्ञानालम्बनं वा॥३८॥

38. Svapna-nidrā-jñānālambanaṁ vā

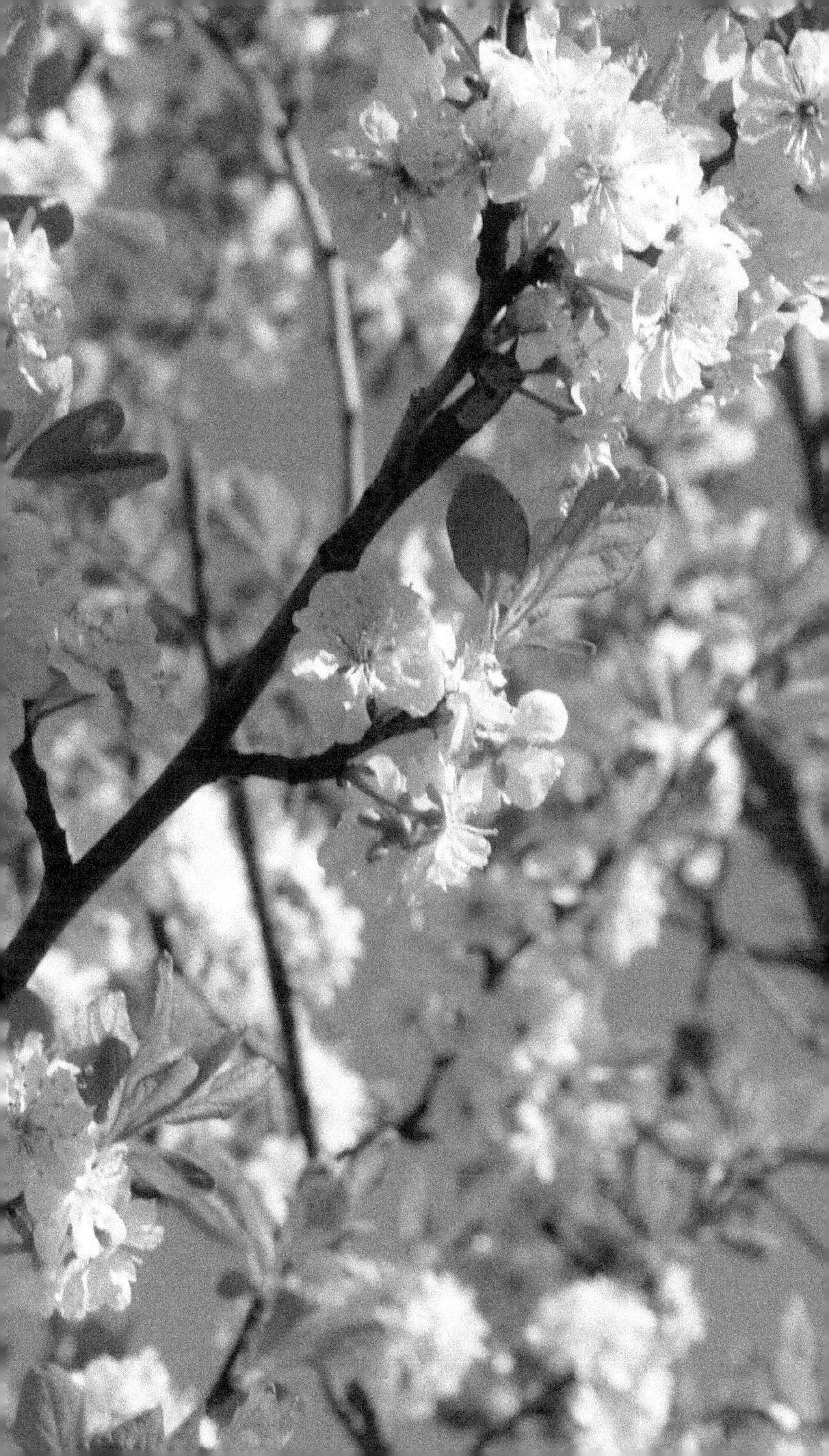

34. *Peace and quiet can be obtained by focusing on breathing.*

Applying breathing exercises (pranayama) is an effective method of taking attention from sensory sensations to presence in the mind, which results in peace and quiet.

35. *When awareness is present at more subtle levels of Consciousness, silence and stability are established.*

As awareness begins to come into contact with consciousness, a characteristic is that sensory activity decreases and an inner stillness arises. This stillness is not dependent on external circumstances. The flow of thoughts decreases and thoughts come only when they fill a necessary need.

36. *When awareness is not bound by sorrow and suffering, inner light can be experienced.*

An inner enlightenment can be experienced in certain states of consciousness. It is not an external physical light that is conveyed via the visual sense, but an inner light that can be experienced as concretely as external light impulses.

37. *Paying attention to someone who is free from*

attachment and desire can lead to awareness becoming focused and present.

Paying attention to someone who is free from attachment and desire can be a help to be able to experience the level of consciousness where there is freedom from attachment and desire. Meeting such a person can mean that this happens spontaneously, but it can also happen at a distance through the invocation in prayer or during meditation. Even reading a text that such a person has written or reading stories about the person in question can affect. Looking at the person in a picture or film can also have such an effect. Therefore, people have always experienced an attraction to saints.

38. If Consciousness is present during sleep or dreamless sleep, this will allow new insights and knowledge and thus stability can be established.

During dream and dreamless sleep, the five senses are not active and thus do not take attention. Thus, awareness can have the opportunity to share knowledge from Consciousness that can provide new insights and contribute to presence in Consciousness. That contributes to stability.

यथाभिमतध्यानाद्वा॥३९॥

39. Yathābhimata-dhyānād vā

परमाणुपरममहत्त्वान्तोऽस्य वशीकारः॥४०॥

40. Paramāṇu-parama-mahattvānto'sya vaśīkāraḥ

क्षीणवृत्तेरभिजातस्येव मणेर्ग्रहीतृग्रहणग्राह्येषु
तत्स्थतदञ्जनता समापत्तिः॥४१॥

41. Kṣīṇa-vṛtter abhijātasyeva maṇer grahītṛ-gra-
haṇa-grāhyeṣu tatstha-tadañjanatā samāpattiḥ

शब्दार्थज्ञानविकल्पैः सङ्कीर्णा सवितर्का
समापत्तिः॥४२॥

42. Tatra śabdārtha-jñāna-vikalpaiḥ saṅkīrṇā savitarkā samāpattiḥ

*39. Also by paying attention to some dear object this
state of consciousness can be achieved.*

*There are many different meditationtechniques that can
be applied to keep focused and present. It can be on an
object, e.g. on a picture of a saint, a flame of fire, on the
function of breathing and exhalation or mentally, on a
sound or a word (a mantra).*

*40. The ability to be consciously present in Conscio-
usness provides the possibility of being present in the
smallest atom up to the infinitely large universe.
When awareness is present in Consciousness there are
no limitations. Then time and space do not constitute
mental limitations.*

*41. Consciousness is like a crystal which is in itself
transparent but which reflects colors from the surroundings. When the senses have ceased to color and bind
the consciousness, the ability to distinguish between the
observer, the ability to observe and the observed arises.*

*When awareness is established in Consciousness the
state of consciousness is no longer colored and bound
by relative existence. Being independent and unaffected
by the relative existence, enables the consciousness to
be able to meet sensory sensations by distinguishing*

*between the observer, the ability to observe and the
observed. Of course, senses and mental activity continue
to act, but a conscious presence is now established that
observes this activity.*

*42. Savitarkā samāpattihis the state of consciousness
in which there is a confusion of the true meaning of a
word, its assumed meaning, and its quality.*

*In the state of consciousness called savitarkā samāpattih
there is uncertainty about the true meaning of a word.
In this state the knowledge of the word is not rooted in
a level of pure Consciousness that is linked to consciousness.*

स्मृतिपरिशुद्धौ स्वरूपशून्येवार्थमात्रनिर्भासा
निर्वितर्का॥४३॥

43. Smṛti-pariśuddhau svarūpa-śūny-
evārtha-mātra-nirbhāsā nirvitarkā

एतयैव सविचारा निर्विचारा च सूक्ष्मविषया
व्याख्याता॥४४॥

44. Etayaiva savicārā nirvicārā ca sūkṣmaviṣayā
vyākhyātā

सूक्ष्मविषयत्वं चालिङ्गपर्यवसानम्॥४५॥

45. Sūkṣma-viṣayatvaṁ cāliṅga-pary-avasānam

ता एव सवीजः समाधिः॥४६॥

46. Tā eva savījaḥ samādhiḥ

निर्विचारवैशारद्येऽध्यात्मप्रसादः॥४७॥

47. Nirvicāra-vaiśāradye 'dhyātma-prasādaḥ

43. Nirvitarka Samadhi is called the state of consciousness which enables true knowledge of an object to be
experienced by the memory being pure and clear and
the attention present without anything distracting it.

When awareness is rooted in Consciousness an object
can be experienced as it is without having it to be jud-
ged through the mind and previous experiences.

44. Savicāra and nirvicāra samadhi are states of consciousness that arise when attention is focused on a subtle
object.

The fact that an object is subtle may mean that it cannot
be experienced by the sense organs or that it cannot be
understood by the intellect. Its existence is beyond the
perceptual capacity of the mind, but can be experienced
on a more subtle level of consciousness.

45. Beyond the experience of the objects' most subtle
state in the manifested nature (prakriti), there is alinga
(the unmanifest).

The relative manifested existence is governed by nature
(prakriti) which is encompassed by (gunas) the three different energies tamas, rajas and sattva. Beyond prakriti
there are alinga ie. the unmanifest.

46. These levels of Consciousness (samādhis) can be seen as basic 'seeds'.

These mentioned levels of Consciousness (samādhis) can be seen as a seed but it has not yet resulted in a fully developed established plant. Awareness is not yet firmly anchored and present in Consciousness.

47. In the state of consciousness called nirvicāra a purification occurs which enables contact with Consciousness.

Through conscious presence and focusing on more subtle levels of consciousness, a purification process begins that result in the removal of stress and tension, both physically and mentally. As a result, the conditions for contact with Consciousness increase.

ऋतम्भरा तत्र प्रज्ञा॥४८॥

48. Ṛtambharā tatra prajñā

श्रुतानुमानप्रज्ञाभ्यामन्यवषिया
वशिषार्थत्वात्॥४९॥

49. Śrutānumāna-prajñābhyām anya-viṣayā
viśeṣārthatvāt

तज्जः संस्कारोऽन्यसंस्कारप्रतबिन्धी॥५०॥

50. Tajjaḥ saṁskāro 'nya-saṁskāra-pratibandhī

तस्यापि निरोधे सर्वनरिोधान्नरिवीजः समाधःि॥५१॥

51. Tasyāpi nirodhe sarva-nirodhān nirvījaḥ samādhiḥ

48. At this level of consciousness, rtambharā prajñā is experienced, which means truth and knowledge.
The truth and knowledge of Consciousness is not relative and not linked to the intellectual conditions of the mind to acquire knowledge and truth. The wisdom of Consciousness is experienced as an obvious insight that comes when one is mature enough to receive it.

49. The knowledge obtained through the level of consciousness in rtambharā does not depend on intellectual inference but comes directly from Consciousness. Intellectual guidance and knowledge from teachers as well as books convey knowledge that is of course also needed in the relative existence, but knowledge and insights that convey spiritual clarity and understanding come directly from Consciousness.

50. When awareness is present in the state of consciousness ritambharā, all sensory impressions are dissipated.

When awareness and Consciousness are united, this state overshadows all other states of consciousness. Sensory sensations and latent senses are then no longer dominant.

51. Once this awareness of Consciousness is established, there is no longer any "seed" to develop. This samādhi means liberation from birth and death.

When awareness of Consciousness is completed and established, there is nothing more to realize. The school of life has ended teaching and then no more lessons are needed and thus no more incarnations in the relative existence. Awareness no longer experiences any dualism in relation to Consciousness.

Chapter 2

SADHANA PADA

To practice yoga exercises

तपःस्वाध्यायेश्वरप्रणिधानानि क्रियायोगः ॥१॥

1. Tapaḥ-svādhyāyeśvara-praṇidhānāni
kriyā-yogaḥ

समाधिभावनार्थः क्लेशतनूकरणार्थश्च ॥२॥

2. Samādhi bhāvanārthaḥ kleśa-tanūkara-ṇārthaś
ca

अविद्यास्मितारागद्वेषाभिनिविशाः पञ्च क्लेशाः ॥३॥

3. Avidyā asmitā-rāga-dveṣābhiniveśāḥ pañca
kleśāḥ

अविद्या क्षेत्रमुत्तरेषां प्रसुप्ततनुविच्छिन्निनोदाराणा
म् ॥४॥

4. Avidyā kṣetram uttareṣāṁ prasupta-tanu-vic-
chinnodārāṇām

अनित्याशुचिदुःखानात्मसु नित्यशुचिसुखात्मख्यातिरि
वदिया ॥५॥

5. Anityāśuci duḥkhānātmasu nitya-śuci-sukhātma
khyātir avidyā

1. Self-discipline, study and surrender to Īśvara (God) enables yoga.

To be focused and ambitious in the practice of spiritual, purifying exercises, and to study holy scriptures, and to surrender to the consciousness of God, is to focus attention on yoga. These are paths for union and identification with Consciousness.

2. This practition brings attention to Samādhi and it minimizes suffering.

As long as states of awareness have the desire for pleasures and sensory objects are dominant and satisfy, life will consist of suffering. The medicine against this is rooted in the Samadhi state of Consciousness.

3. Kleśāh(suffering) is due to avidyā (ignorance) and results in asmitā (egoism), rāga (bondage), dvesa (aversion) and abhiniveśah(death anxiety).

As long as awareness is bound to the mind, avidyā prevails, ie. There is ignorance of identity with Consciousness. In this state of awareness, the ego dominates. As the will and desires of the ego do not always correspond to the reality of the present, conflict and suffering arise. The will and desires of the ego also come into conflict with an imagined future. Because the ego sees its existence limited to time and space, death is the worst that can occur, which causes death anxiety as it means the end of the ego.

4. Avidyā (ignorance) is the cause of suffering which can be dormant, diminishing or active and increasing.

When consciousness is rooted in the mind, the life situation shifts between happiness and joy as well as suffering. As there are periods of happiness and joy, suffering still remains latent.

5. Ignorance is to identify with non-ātma (non-self) instead of ātma (Self) and to confuse the temporary with the eternal, the unclean with the pure, and suffering as enjoyable.

The state of ignorance is characterized by mental confusion and is an illusory state. To be identified with non-ātma (non-self) instead of ātma (Self) means to be anchored in the mind instead of Consciousness.

दृग्दर्शनशक्त्योरेकात्मतेवास्मिता॥६॥

6. Dṛg-darśana-śaktyor ekātmatevāsmitā

सुखानुशयी रागः॥७॥

7. Sukhānuśayī rāgaḥ

दुःखानुशयी द्वेषः॥८॥

8. Duḥkhānuśayī dveṣaḥ

स्वरसवाही विदुषोऽपि तथारूढोऽभिनिवेशः॥९॥

9. Svarasavāhī viduṣo 'pi tathā rūḍho 'bhiniveśaḥ

ते परतिप्रसवहेयाः सूक्ष्माः॥१०॥

10. Te pratiprasava-heyāḥ sūkṣmāḥ

*6. Asmitā (individuality, egoism) arises when the mind
and intellect, thinks itself to be ātma (the Self or Consciousness), this confusion then becomes an obstacle to the
experience of Consciousness.*

*When awareness is rooted in an identity that has been
created by the mind, intellect and ego, this identity
becomes relative and limited. Individuality arises
through the assumption that this relative and limited
state of awareness is the real self. The real self is in fact
not relative and limited but absolute and eternally pure
Consciousness.*

7. Bondage arises through desire.

*Some desires can bind awareness to the mind and beco-
me an obstacle to the experience of Consciousness.*

8. Out of suffering arises aversion.

*An ongoing suffering often creates a negative mood and
low energy.*

*9. Death anxiety and the need to cling to life are present
in all of us, even in the wise.*

Anxiety about death and the will to live are strongly

established in every human being. If breathing ceases, there will automatically be death anxiety to protect life.

10. These obstacles disappear when awareness is rooted in Consciousness.

Suffering and ignorance exist as long as awareness is rooted in the mind. To be present in Consciousness means to no longer be bound by suffering and ignorance.

ध्यानहेयास्तद्वृत्तयः॥११॥

11. Dhyāna-heyās-tad-vṛttayaḥ

क्लेशमूलः कर्माशयो दृष्टादृष्टजन्मवेदनीयः॥१२॥

12. Kleśa-mūlaḥ karmāśayo dṛṣṭādṛṣṭa-janmave-
daniyaḥ

सति मूले तद्विपाको जात्यायुर्भोगाः॥१३॥

13. Sati mūle tad-vipāko jāty-āyur-bhogāḥ

ते ह्लादपरितापफलाः पुण्यापुण्यहेतुत्वात्॥१४॥

14. Te hlāda-paritāpa-phalāḥ puṇyāpuṇya-hetutvāt

परिणामतापसंस्कारदुःखैर्गुणवृत्तविरोधाच्च दुःखमेव
सर्वं विवेकिनः॥१५॥

15. Pariṇāma-tāpa-saṁskāra-duḥkhair guṇa-vṛt-
ti-virodhāc ca duḥkham eva sarvaṁ vivekinaḥ

11. To anchor awareness in Consciousness to get rid of anxiety and suffering can be done through meditation.

Allowing attention to be present in Consciousness through meditation can be a way to get rid of anxiety and stress that causes suffering.

12. Karmāśaya (karma) are experiences that are latent and expressed in action in this life or in future life.

What has been done cannot be undone, therefore life cannot be in any other way than it is right now. The law of karma is relentless and cannot be negotiated away. Sooner or later comes the effect of an act. This applies to both an individual and to a collective level. At the level of the mind, one may think that "no one knows" or "one has soon forgotten". But everything that happens is registered and not forgotten, by the observer at the level of Consciousness.

13. As long as there is stored karma, this karma will manifest itself in the form of birth and a life cycle of actions.

The stored quota of karma (the bank of experience) wants to manifest itself in a life situation and therefore there is a reason for birth. All desires that have not been allowed to manifest themselves are waiting for an opportunity to become established.

14. Good or bad karma results in happiness and suffering respectively.

Karma is like seeds that are sown in soil and begin to germinate into a plant. The plant can become a thorny shrub or a beautiful flower depending on the conditions of the seed.

15. He who observes sees that all relative experiences lead to suffering and anxiety no matter which of the three gunas dominates, and that enjoyable moods are transient.

हेयं दुःखमनागतम् ॥१६॥

16. Heyaṁ duḥkha manāgatam

दरष्टृद्दृश्ययोः संयोगो हेयहेतुः ॥१७॥

17. Draṣṭṛ-dṛśyayoḥ saṁyogo heya-hetuḥ

प्रकाशक्रियास्थतिशीलं भूतेन्द्रियात्मकं
भोगापवर्गार्थं दृश्यम् ॥१८॥

18. Prakāśa-kriyā-sthiti-śīlaṁ bhūtendriyāt-makaṁ
bhogāpavargārthaṁ dṛśyam

विशेषाविशेषलङ्गिमात्रालङ्गिगानि गुणपर्वाणि ॥१९॥

19. Viśeṣāviśeṣa-liṅgamātrāliṅgāni guṇa-parvāṇi

दरष्टा दृशमिात्रः शुद्धोऽपि परत्ययानुपश्यः ॥२०॥

20. Draṣṭā dṛśimātraḥ śuddho 'pi pratyayā-nu-
paśyaḥ

*16. Suffering that has not yet manifested can be avoided.
Being rooted in the mind means that both good and
bad karma affect the presence in the present. Karma
manifests itself as impulses that want to become aware
and manifested. He who is rooted in Consciousness has
the opportunity to be unaffected by these impulses and
can therefore avoid the consequences of karma.
17. The cause of suffering is that the observer identifies
with what is observed.*

*As long as the observer identifies with the observation,
ie. with the mind and with the senses, there is duality
and thus a prerequisite for suffering. When the observer
is rooted in Consciousness, there is no longer any duality
and thus there is no conflict that can create suffering.*

*18. What can be observed is the relative existence of the
five elements and the energies of tamas, rajas and sat-
vas. The purpose of its existence is to provide experiences that lead to liberation.*

*The purpose of experiences that lead to liberation is to
be liberated from being enslaved by the mind and its
desires, in order to be present in the absolute eternal
existence of Consciousness.*

19. The three gunas affect awareness with impulses or

sensations that can be subtle or gross, perceptible or unconscious.

Some impulses from the three gunas can be understood intellectually and can be put into words, while others are perceived on a subtle emotional level.

20. Pure Consciousness is untouched as it witnesses the mind and the senses.

When awareness is anchored in Consciousness what is happening in the present is witnessed and then freedom arises to decide whether the sensory sensations are to be manifested or not. This means that the mind cannot enslave Consciousness. Only then does real freedom and understanding arise such as; that the mind no longer alone affects the event.

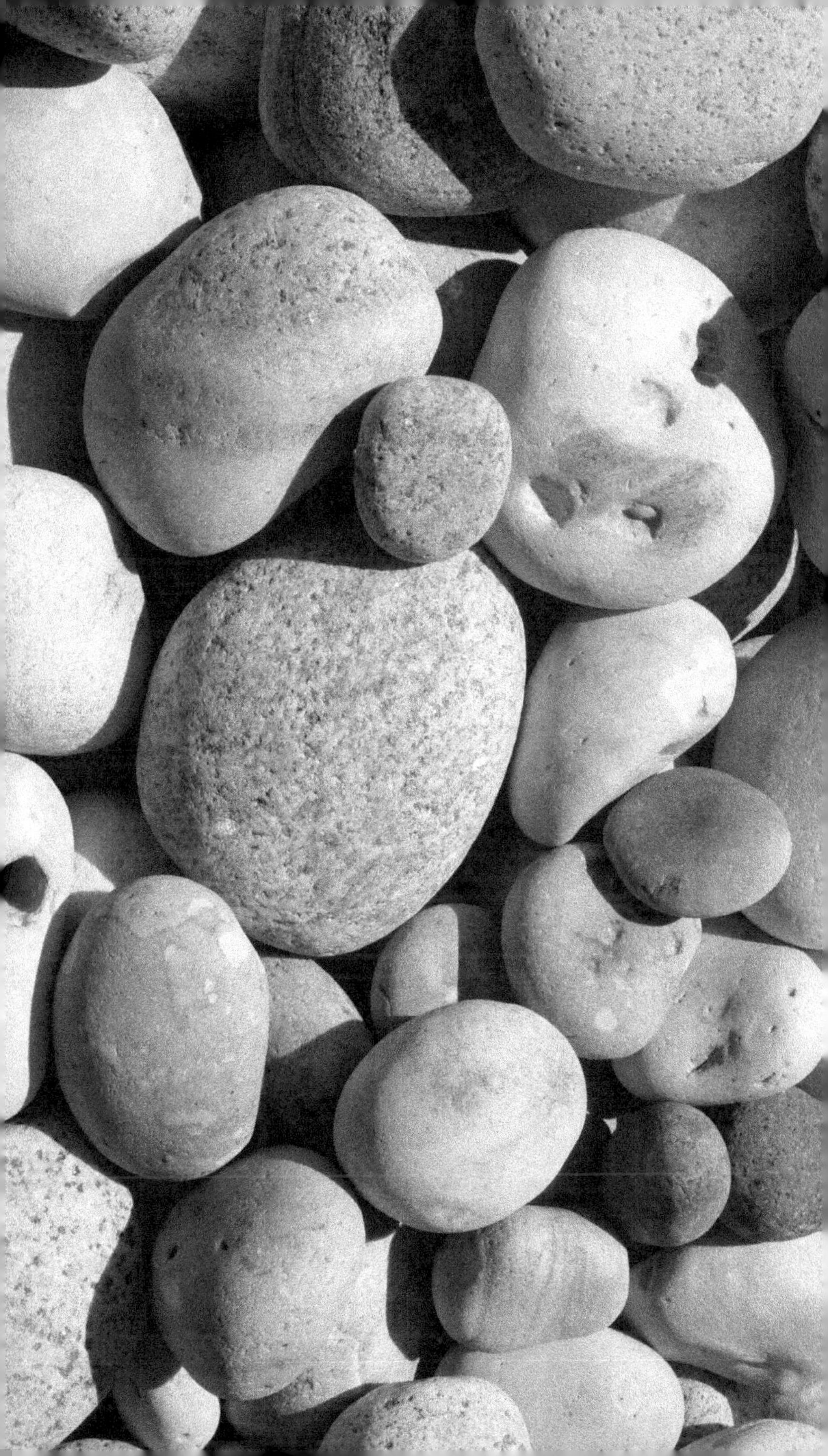

तदर्थ एव दृश्यस्यात्मा॥२१॥

21. Tad-artha eva dṛśyasyātmā

कृतार्थं प्रति नष्टमप्यनष्टं
तदन्यसाधारणत्वात्॥२२॥

22. Kṛtārthaṁ prati naṣṭam apy anaṣṭaṁ
tad-anya-sādhāraṇatvāt

स्वस्वामिशक्त्योः स्वरूपोपलब्धहितुः संयोगः॥२३॥

23. Sva-svāmi-śaktyoḥ svarūpopalabdhi-hetuḥ
saṁyogaḥ

तस्य हेतुरविद्या॥२४॥

24. Tasya hetur avidyā

तदभावात्संयोगाभावो हानं तद्दृशेः कैवल्यम्॥२५॥

25. Tad-abhāvāt saṁyogābhāvo hānaṁ tad dṛśeḥ
kaivalyam

21. The manifested exists for Consciousness (ātmān).

The world and relative existence exist as mental sensory sensations for consciousness.

22. The mental sensations are not real to the one who is present in the Consciousness, while they are reality to the one who is bound to the mind.

Life is experienced differently depending on the level of awareness on which the experience is based.

23. When the observer observes what is observed, the true identity of both the observer and the observed is experienced.

When awareness is present in Consciousness, ie. the observer, the true identity of both the observer and the observed is revealed.

24. Identifying with what is observed depends on ignorance.

As long as one identifies with body and mind, reality is obscured by ignorance. It is not an intellectual ignorance but an experiential ignorance, ie. it is about lack of experience in identifying with the observer. .

25. When the identification with the observer becomes conscious, the ignorance disappears and the awareness is liberated and enlightened.

To be consciously present in Consciousness means that everything unreal and false disappears and that only the absolute pure Consciousness is conscious. This state of awareness is usually called the state of enlightenment or liberation.

वविकख्यातरिवप्िलवा हानोपायः॥२६॥

26. Viveka-khyātir aviplavā hānopāyaḥ

तस्य सप्तधा परान्तभूमिः परज्ञा॥२७॥

27. Tasya saptadhā prānta-bhūmiḥ prajñā

योगाङ्गानुष्ठानादशुद्धक्िषये
ज्ञानदीप्तरिवविकख्यातेः॥२८॥

28. Yogāṅgānuṣṭhānād aśuddhi-kṣaye jñāna-dīptir
ā viveka-khyāteḥ

यमनयिमासनप्राणायामप्रत्याहारधारणाध्यानसमाधयो
ऽष्टावङ्गानि॥२९॥

29. Yama-niyamāsana-prāṇāyāma-pra-
tyāhāra-dhāraṇā-dhyāna-samādhayo'ṣṭāv aṅgāni

26. Being constantly anchored in Consciousness enables the ignorance to disappear.

To be constantly aware of Consciousness means that every illusions and that all ignorance do not have the opportunity to affect consciousness.

27. Seven ways can be applied to become aware of Consciousness.

The seven paths can be applied either individually or they can be combined.

28. By practicing these exercises, impurities can be removed and this increases the possibility of being able to be aware of Consciousness and thus have access to the ability to distinguish the real from the unreal.

Practicing these exercises does not automatically guarantee that the awareness can be aware of Consciousness, but the conditions will be better.

29. The eight limbs of yoga are;

yama - properties that provide purity and harmony
niyama - rules of life that provide purity and harmony
āsana - postures

prānāyāma - breathing exercises

pratyāhāra - to divert attention from the objects of the mind

dhāranā - conscious presence beyond the mind

dhyāna - meditation

samādhi - conscious presence in Consciousness

These eight limbs constitute the eightfold path "ashtanga yoga".

अहिंसासत्यास्तेयब्रह्मचर्यापरिग्रिहा यमाः॥३०॥

30. Ahiṁsā satyāsteya-brahmacaryāparigrahā
yamāḥ

जातिदेशकालसमयानवच्छन्निाः सार्वभौमा
महाव्रतम्॥३१॥

31. Jāti-deśa-kāla-samayānavacchinnāḥ sār-
vabhaumā mahā-vratam

शौचसन्तोषतपःस्वाध्यायेश्वरप्रणिधानानि
नियमाः॥३२॥

32. Śauca-santoṣa-tapaḥ-svādhyāyeśvara-praṇid-
hānāni niyamāḥ

*30. Yama - qualities that provide inner purity, peace
and harmony.*

ahimsā - non-violence
satya - to stick to the truth
asteya - absence of greed
brahmacarya - abstinence (celibacy)
aparigrahāh - not to have a desire to own

*Being aware of, and living by, these qualities or rules
lays the foundation for a life of peace and harmony.*

*31. These yamas are universal laws that are not limited
by time, place, environment, or the prevailing situation.
Yamas are laws rooted in universal wisdom.*

32. Niyama - the five rules of life.

śauca - purity
santosa - contentment
tapas - self-discipline
svādhyāya - self-study
īśvarapranidhānā - surrender to God

*Niyama's rules of life are there to facilitate a conscious
presence in the Consciousness. To keep body and soul
pure through exercise, self-discipline and healthy food,*

*to be content with what is and to read scriptures that
contain wisdom, this provides the best conditions for
being able to surrender to God.*

वितिर्कबाधने परतपिक्षभावनम्॥३३॥
33. Vitarka-bādhane pratipakṣa-bhāvanam

वितिर्का हसिादयः कृतकारतिानुमोदतिा
लोभक्रोधमोहपूर्वका मृदुमध्याधमिात्रा
दुःखाज्ञानानन्तफला इति परतपिक्षभावनम्॥३४॥
34. Vitarkā hiṁsādayaḥ kṛta-kāritānumoditā
lobha-krodha-moha-pūrvakā mṛdu-madhyād-
himātrā duḥkhājñānānanta-phalā iti pratipakṣa-bhāvanam

अहिसिापरतषि्ठायां तत्सन्ननिधौ वैरत्यागः॥३५॥
35, Ahiṁsā-pratiṣṭhāyāṁ tat-sannidhau vai-
ra-tyāgaḥ

सत्यपरतषि्ठायां क्रयिाफलाश्रयत्वम्॥३६॥
36. Satya-pratiṣṭhāyāṁ kriyā-phalāśrayatvam

असतेयपरतषि्ठायां सर्वरत्नोपसथानम्॥३७॥
37. Asteya-pratiṣṭhāyāṁ sarva-ratnopasthānam

33. When awareness is rooted in negative and bad thoughts these can be neutralized if opposite thoughts become conscious instead.

Negative and bad thoughts are generated through the dysfunctional ego. By being rooted in Consciousness these thoughts can not exist and thoughts based on wisdom become conscious instead.

34. Negative and bad thoughts, feelings, and actions, whether caused by greed, anger, or confusion, can be minor, moderate, or intense. They always lead to suffering and ignorance and therefore it is necessary to pay attention to the opposite.

Paying attention to the opposite means paying attention to Consciousness, whish is not limited by the ego.

35. As awareness is rooted in non-violence (ahimsā), the environment will also cease to be hostile.

The energy that a person present in Consciousness radiates affects everyone in the environment more strongly than the energy that emanates from the one who is rooted in the mind.

36. Being rooted in truth (satya) gives the best result and the fruit of action arises without effort.

He who is established in Consciousness becomes a tool for Consciousness and there is then no other alternative to satya, ie. truth. Action is then no longer an action that has a selfish motive, the action is motivated for the good of the whole. The action is performed without resistance and struggle and is therefore perceived as effortless.

37. Being honest and refraining from stealing (asteya), enables all the wealth needed to arise.

He who is honest creates karma, which means that he gets access to what is needed in the current life situation.

ब्रह्मचर्यप्रतिष्ठायां वीर्यलाभः ॥३८॥

38. Brahmacarya-pratiṣṭhāyāṁ vīrya-lābhaḥ

अपरिग्रहस्थैर्ये जन्मकथन्तासम्बोधः ॥३९॥

39. Aparigraha-sthairye janma-kathantā-sambod-

haḥ

शौचात्स्वाङ्गजुगुप्सा परैरसंसर्गः ॥४०॥

40. Śaucāt svāṅga-jugupsā parair asaṁsargaḥ

सत्त्वशुद्धसौमनस्यैकाग्र्येन्द्रियजयात्मदर्शनयोग्
यत्वानि च ॥४१॥

41. Sattvaśuddhi-saumanasyaikāgryendriya-jayāt-

ma-darśana-yogyatvāni ca

सन्तोषादनुत्तमसुखलाभः ॥४२॥

42. Santoṣādanuttamasukhalābhaḥ

38. Being established in sexual abstinence (brahmacarya) provides spiritual energy.

The desire for sexual pleasure is a strong energy that takes attention to body and mind. Sexual gratification increases sexual desire. Thus, the awareness of Consciousness can be lost and the spiritual energy that arises when this association is conscious can then also be lost. Being free from sexual desire enables more easyly the presence of Consciousness.

39. Not having a desire to own (aparigraha) gives knowledge of existence.

The desire for power and wealth is a strong energy that binds awareness to the mind. This negative energy arises from the mind through the greed of the ego and is the root of many of humanity's problems. Mastering greed provides access to knowledge and wisdom.

40. When inner purity (śaucā) is achieved, this leads to independence from one's own body and indifference to other bodies.

As the experience of inner purification dominates awareness one's own body is no longer perceived as something with which one identifies and other bodies are no longer perceived as attractive.

41. Through sattvic purification peace and harmony arise, the ability to be consciously present, control of the mind, and the opportunity to experience Consciousness. The sattvic purification occurs when sattva dominates tamas and rajas. In this pure state are the best spiritual conditions.

42. Satisfaction (santosā) brings the highest happiness. To be established in the pure state, ie. being consciously present in Consciousness gives total contentment and the highest happiness.

कायेन्द्रियसिद्धिरशुद्धिक्षयात्तपसः ॥४३॥

43. Kāyendriya-siddhir aśuddhi-kṣayāt tapasaḥ

स्वाध्यायादिष्टदेवतासम्प्रयोगः ॥४४॥

44. Svādhyāyād iṣṭa-devatā samprayogaḥ

समाधिसिद्धिरीश्वरप्रणिधानात् ॥४५॥

45. Samādhi-siddhir īśvara-praṇidhānāt

स्थिरसुखमासनम् ॥४६॥

46. Sthira-sukham āsanam

प्रयत्नशैथिल्यानन्तसमापत्तिभ्याम् ॥४७॥

47. Prayatna-śaithilyānanta samāpattibhyām

43. *Through spiritual exercises (tapas) impurities are removed and purity is achieved in body and soul. Spiritual exercises can be meditation (yoga dhyana), postures (yoga asana) or breathing exercises (yoga pranayama).*

44. *Studying spiritual scriptures (svādhyāyā) can lead to union with the divine.*

When attention is directed to a scripture that describes the union with the divine Consciousness, a desire may arise to experience this, which can then also result in experience of this union (yoga).

45. *The result of devotion to and union with the Divine Consciousness (īśvarapranidhānā) is samādhi.*

This level of awareness that results in yoga or samādhi means a state of Consciousness has been achieved that is complete, ie. there is nothing more to look for.

46. *The physical position (āsana) should be stable but still comfortable.*

By being consciously present in the body, the association with Consciousness is facilitated. Mastering the lotus position (padmāsana) provides a stable and comfortable position that is suitable for meditation.

*47. Through a relaxed attitude awareness of Conscio-
usness can be established and thus eternity can become
conscious.*

*When awareness is no longer present in mental activity
the eternity can become conscious. When the time- and
space-bound mind no longer controls awareness, reality
can manifest itself. Being in a relaxed state of awareness
can be helpful for this process.*

ततो द्वन्द्वानभिघातः ॥४८॥

48. Tato dvandvānabhighātaḥ

तस्मिन्सति श्वासप्रश्वासयोर्गतविच्छेदः
प्राणायामः ॥४९॥

49. Tasmin sati śvāsa-prasvāsayor gati-vicchedaḥ
prāṇāyāmaḥ

वाह्याभ्यन्तरस्तम्भवृत्तिः देशकालसङ्ख्याभिः
परिदृष्टो दीर्घसूक्ष्मः ॥५०॥

50. Bāhyābhyantara-stambha-vṛttir deśakāla-saṅk-
hyābhiḥ paridṛṣṭo dīrghasūkṣmaḥ

वाह्याभ्यन्तरविषयाक्षेपी चतुर्थः ॥५१॥

51. Bāhyābhyantara-viṣayākṣepī caturthaḥ

ततः क्षीयते प्रकाशावरणम् ॥५२॥

52. Tataḥ kṣīyate prakāśāvaraṇam

48. When awareness is rooted in Consciousness, the duality of sensory perceptions can be observed and thus they no longer cause bother.

Being able to observe the duality of sensory perceptions means that it is possible to separate the real from the unreal and thus not become a victim of their delusions.

49. By practicing breathing exercises (prānāyāma), which involves conscious presence in inhalation and exhalation, the breathing activity is calmed.

Prānā is the subtle energy that is manifested in the relative existence, ie. life energy. Through breathing exercises, prana can be experienced will then provide harmony and energy.

50. Breathing (at pranayama) changes depending on time and place and in intensity, it can be experienced as inhalation, exhalation or temporary cessation, it can be experienced as prolonged or short.

In pranayama, breathing is experienced in three different phases inhalation, exhalation and cessation of breathing, as long as consciousness is present at the level of the respiratory function.

51. The fourth type of pranayama goes beyond the inner and outer spheres.

When this type of pranayama is performed, the conscious presence can leave the level of the respiratory function to the autonomous system, to be aware in Consciousness.

52. In this way, the veil that obscures the inner light can be removed.

The inner light is not a light from any outer object such as the sun or a lamp, but the light from within. This light can be experienced without the visual sense being involved and is experienced as lightning from within.

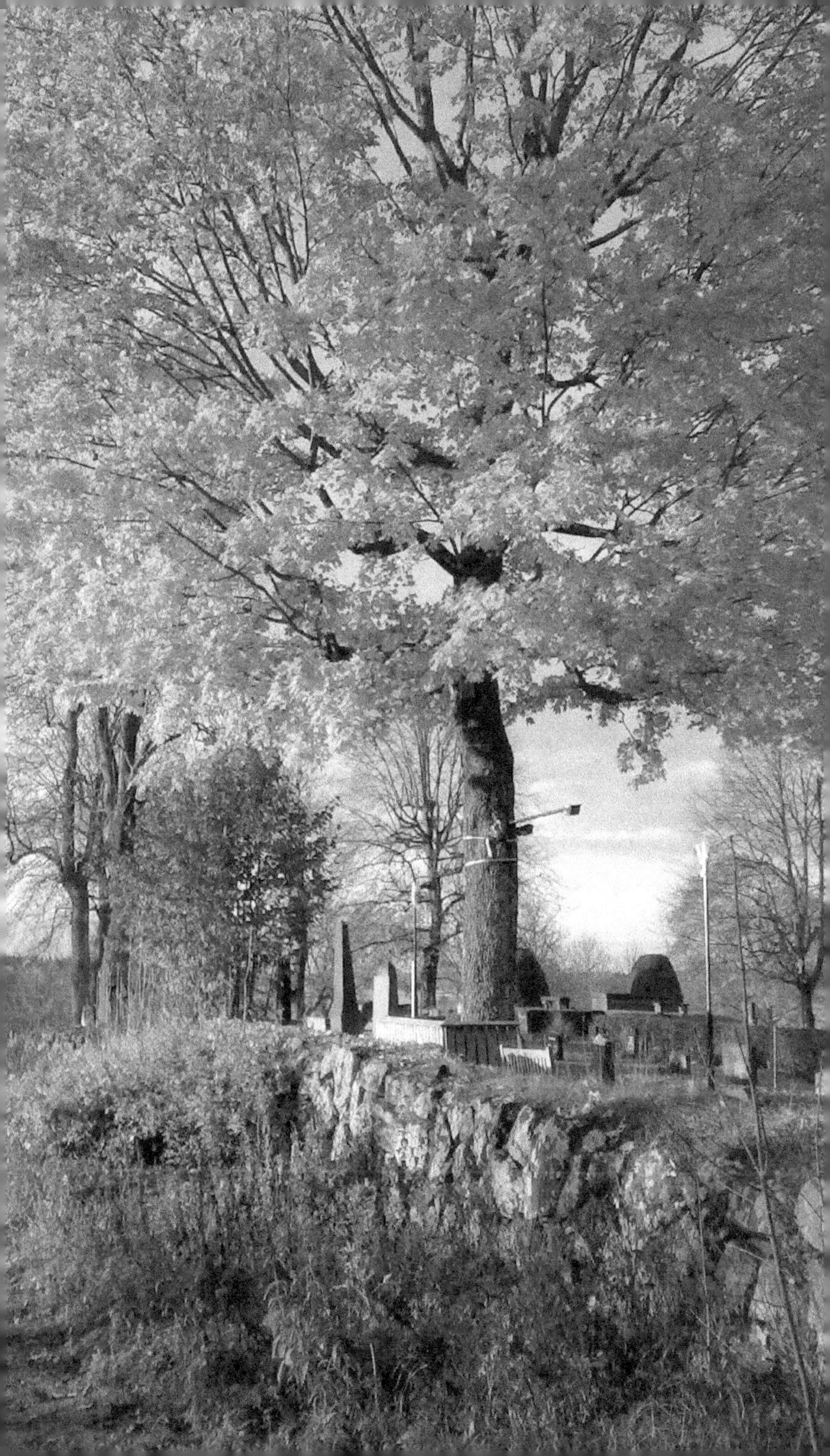

धारणासु च योग्यता मनसः॥५३॥

53. Dhāraṇāsu ca yogyatā manasaḥ

स्वविषयासम्प्रयोगे चित्तस्य स्वरूपानुकार
इवेन्द्रियाणां प्रत्याहारः॥५४॥

54. Sva-viṣayāsamprayoge cittasya sva-
rūpānukāra ivendriyāṇāṁ pratyāhāraḥ

ततः परमा वश्यतेन्द्रियाणाम्॥५५॥

55. Tataḥ paramā vaśyatendriyāṇām

53. *Then awareness becomes consciously present (dhāranā).*

This state of consciousness involves presence in the body, mind and Consciousness.

54. *When the senses is drawn away from awareness, this is called pratyāhāra.*

This state of consciousness is characterized by the absence of sensory activity such as thoughts, emotions and impressions from the sense organs.

55. *This state of consciousness involves spontaneous mastery of the mind.*

Trying to control the mind with the help of the intellect is doomed to fail. By releasing the anchorage in the intellect and being present in Consciousness, the mind acquires a subordinate function and then does not dominate awareness.

Chapter 3

VIBHUTI PADA

Spiritual powers and abilities

देशबन्धश्चित्तस्य धारणा॥१॥

1. Deśa-bandhaś cittasya dhāraṇā

तत्र प्रत्ययैकतानता ध्यानम्॥२॥

2. Tatra pratyayaikatānatā dhyānam

तदेवार्थमात्रनिर्भासं स्वरूपशून्यमिव समाधिः॥३॥

3. Tad evārthamātra-nirbhāsaṁ svarūpa-śūnyami-
va samādhiḥ

त्रयमेकत्र संयमः॥४॥

4. Trayam ekatra saṁyamaḥ

तज्जयात्प्रज्ञालोकः॥५॥

5. Taj-jayāt prajñālokaḥ

तस्य भूमिषु विनियोगः॥६॥

6. Tasya bhūmiṣu viniyogaḥ

1. To be present is dhāranā.

To concentrate on something is dhāranā.

2. To allow awareness to flow towards a specific object is called meditation (dhyāna).

To be present both in the now and simultaneously let the attention be directed towards the object of meditation means that an association with the object of meditation can take place.

3. When awareness can be reconciled with and is undisturbed by the meditation object, the state of consciousness, samādhi, arises.

If the senses don´t distract when consciousness is united with the object of meditation, awareness of Consciousness can arise. This condition is called yoga or samādhi.

4. When these three (dhāranā, dhyāna and samādhi) work together, samyama arises.

Samyama is a condition that can be temporary or permanent.

5. In this state of consciousness there is access to the light of intuitive knowledge.

Intuitive knowledge does not come from e.g. via a book or a teacher but from within and it comes "like lightning from a clear sky". This knowledge does not need to be valued and questioned intellectually.

6. Its (samyama) application takes place via various steps.

Samyama does not arise through intellectual understanding but through practical application and practice.

तरयमन्तरङ्गं पूर्वेभ्यः ॥७॥

7. Trayam antaraṅgaṁ pūrvebhyaḥ

तदपि वहिरङ्गं निर्वीजस्य ॥८॥

8. Tad api vahir-aṅgaṁ nirvījasya

व्युत्थाननिरोधसंस्कारयोरभिभिवप्रादुर्भावौ
निरोधक्षणचित्तान्वयो निरोधपरिणामः ॥९॥

9. Vyutthāna-nirodha-saṁskāray-
or-abhibha-va-prādurbhāvau nirodha-kṣaṇa-cittān-
vayo nirodha-pariṇāmaḥ

तस्य प्रशान्तवाहिता संस्कारात् ॥१०॥

10. Tasya praśānta-vāhitā saṁskārat

सर्वार्थतैकाग्रतयोः क्षयोदयौ चित्तस्य
समाधिपरिणामः ॥११॥

11. Sarvārthataikāgratayoḥ kṣayodayau cittasya
samādhi-pariṇāmaḥ

*7. These three (dhāranā, dhyāna and samādhi) affect
more directly than the five previously described paths;
(yama, niyama, āsana, prānāyāma and pratyāhāra).*

*Once samyama is established, the state of consciousness
yoga can be experienced, while yama, niyama, āsana,
prānāyāma, and pratyāhāra are different paths that can
lead to yoga.*

*8. But even these three (dhāranā, dhyāna and samādhi)
are inferior to the highest level of samādhi.*

*Samādhi can be experienced as inner peace and tran-
quility, but absent of sensory experiences. The highest
state of samādhi occurs when awareness is completely
absorbed in Consciousness. From this samādhi there is
no return back to the ignorance where the mind rules
and where identification with the mind takes place.*

*9. Nirodha parināmah is a state where awareness is
present in ongoing sensory experiences and in vanishing
sensory experiences, thus to be established in silence and
stillness without sensory sensations.*

*Nirodha parināmah is the transition from being bound
by sensory senses to being an observer of what is happening in the present.*

10. Then a flowing, calm and peaceful state of awareness arises.

When sensory experiences cease, there are no conflicts, no resistance, and no duality. When all resistance is gone, a flow of peace, well-being and silence is experienced.

11. The state of consciousness samādhi parināmah is characterized by the experience of unity. All disturbances are then gone.

Samādhi parināmah means that all division and duality is gone and has been replaced by wholeness and unity.

ततः पुनः शान्तोदितौ तुल्यप्रत्ययौ
चित्तस्यैकाग्रतापरिणामः ॥१२॥

12. Tataḥ punaḥ śāntoditau tulya-pratyayau cit-
tasyaikāgratā-pariṇāmaḥ

एतेन भूतेन्द्रियेषु धर्मलक्षणावस्थापरिणामा
व्याख्याताः ॥१३॥

13. Etena bhūtendriyeṣu dharma-lakṣaṇā-vast-
hā-pariṇāmā vyākhyātāḥ

शान्तोदिताव्यपदेश्यधर्मानुपाती धर्मी ॥१४॥

14. Śāntoditāvyapadeśya-dharmānupātī dharmī

क्रमान्यत्वं परिणामान्यत्वे हेतुः ॥१५॥

15. Kramānyatvaṁ pariṇāmānyatve hetuḥ

12. Ekāgratā parināma is a state of awareness which means that the conscious presence is bound to a constant flow of sensory sensations both from the past and from the present.

As long as this state of awareness is present, it means a constant bond to the mind and sensory sensations both from the past, present and future.

13. The state of awareness changes depending on characteristics, character, and the function of the body and the sense organs.

How awareness perceives life in the present depends, among other things, on the body and the function and properties of the mind.

14. All manifested objects are characterized by the fact that they change and have a past, a being in the present, and a future.

Objects in space and time are constantly changing and are bound to the principle of the maintenance and degradation of creation.

15. The cause of the changes are the laws of nature that govern evolution.

The relative manifested existence is governed by certain given laws of nature.

In the following sutras, Patanjali gives various suggestions on how it is possible to influence the laws of nature and the manifested relative existence, and how it is possible to obtain so-called, siddhis (occult forces). Some yogis consider it reprehensible to use these siddhis as they draw attention to the mind and ego and away from the divine Consciousness. In sutra 38, Patanjali says that they are obstacles to achieving samādhi.

परिणामत्रयसंयमादतीतानागतज्ञानम्॥१६॥

16. Pariṇāma-traya-saṁyamād atītānāgata-jñā-
nam

शब्दार्थप्रत्यायानामितरेतराध्यासात्सङ्करस्तत्प्रवि
भागसंयमात्सर्वभूतरुतज्ञानम्॥१७॥

17. Śabdārtha-pratyayānām itaretarādhyāsāt
saṁkaras tat-pravibhāga-saṁyamāt sarva-bhū-
ta-ruta-jñānam

संस्कारसाक्षात्करणात्पूर्वजातिज्ञानम्॥१८॥

18. Saṁskāra-sākṣātkaraṇāt pūrva-jātijñānam

प्रत्ययस्य परचित्तिज्ञानम्॥१९॥

19. Pratyayasya para-citta-jñānam

न च तत्सालम्बनं तस्याविषयीभूतत्वात्॥२०॥

20. Na ca tat sālambanaṁ tasyāviṣayī-bhū-tatvāt

कायरूपसंयमात्तद्ग्राह्यशक्तिस्तिम्भे चक्षुःप्रकाशा
सम्प्रयोगेऽन्तर्धानम्॥२१॥

21. Kāya-rūpa-saṁyamāt tad-grāhya-śakti-stam-
bhe cakṣuḥ-prakāśāsamprayoge 'ntardhānam

एतेन शदाद्यतधारनमुक्तमः ॥ २२॥

22. Etena śabdādy antardhānam uktamḥ

16. *By practicing the samyama on the three changing states (nirodha, samādhi and ekāgrata), knowledge of the past and of the future can be obtained.*

17. *A sound, its meaning, and idea are mixed. By making samyama on each part separately, this results in that, the sounds of all living beings can be understood.*

18. *By performing samyama on past experiences, knowledge of past lives can be obtained.*

19. *Doing samyama on mental images that arise consciously can provide knowledge about the minds of others.*

20. *The purpose of practicing samyama on the minds of others is not the content but the quality and feeling experienced.*

21. *By making samyama on the shape of a body, the contact between an observer's eye and the light of the body can be broken and it can then become invisible.*

22. *The result is also that sounds etc., cease to be heard.*

सोपक्रमं नरिुपक्रमं च कर्म
तत्संयमादपरान्तज्ञानमरिष्टेभ्यो वा॥२२॥
23. Sopakramaṁ nirupakramaṁ ca karma
tat-saṁyamād aparānta-jñānam ariṣṭebhyo vā

मैत्र्यादिषु बलानि॥२३॥
24. Maitryādiṣu balāni

बलेषु हस्तबिलादीनि॥२४॥
25. Baleṣu hasti-balādīni

परवृत्त्यालोकन्यासात्सूक्ष्मव्यवहतिविप्रकृष्टज्ञान
म्॥२५॥
26. Pravṛtty-āloka-nyāsāt sūkṣma-vyavahita-vi-
prakṛṣṭa-jñānam

भुवनज्ञानं सूर्ये संयमात्॥२६॥
27. Bhuvana-jñānaṁ sūrye saṁyamāt

चन्द्रे ताराव्यूहज्ञानम्॥२७॥
28. Candre tārā-vyūha-jñānam

23. By performing samyama on two kinds of karma;
the active and the dormant, the time of the moment of
death can be experienced.

24. Practicing samyama in kindness, compassion, and
happiness can mean that these qualities are obtained.

25. By practicing the samyama on the strength of an
elephant, such strength can be obtained.

26. To practice samyama on the inner light, knowledge
of the subtle, the hidden, and the distant object can be
obtained.

27. By doing samyama on the sun, knowledge of the
solar system can be obtained.

28. Practicing samyama on the moon, can provide
knowledge of star systems.

ध्रुवे तद्गतिज्ञानम्॥२८॥

29. Dhruve tad-gati-jñānam

नाभिचक्रे कायव्यूहज्ञानम्॥२९॥

30. Nābhi-cakre kāya-vyūhajñānam

कण्ठकूपे क्षुत्पिपासानिवृत्तिः॥३०॥

31. Kaṇṭha-kūpe kṣut-pipāsā-nivṛttiḥ

कूर्मनाड्यां स्थैर्यम्॥३१॥

32. Kūrma-nāḍyāṁ sthairyam

मूर्धज्योतिषि सिद्धदर्शनम्॥३२॥

33. Mūrdha-jyotiṣi siddha-darśanam

प्रातिभाद्वा सर्वम्॥३३॥

34. Prātibhād vā sarvam

हृदये चित्तसंवित्॥३४॥

35. Hṛdaye citta-saṁvit

29. *By practicing the samyama on the pole star, this gives knowledge of the movements of the stars.*

30. *To make samyama on the navel, knowledge of the structure of the body can be obtained.*

31. *Through samyama on the trachea, hunger and thirst can be quenched.*

32. *Practicing samyama on the bronchial tubes (kūr-ma-nādi) provides silence.*

33. *By practicing samyama on the light in the head enlightened persons (siddhas) may be experienced.*

34. *Practicing samyama on intuition (prātibhā), means that everything can be understood.*

35. *By practicing samyama on the heart, knowledge of the mind can be obtained.*

सत्त्वपुरुषयोरत्यन्तासङ्कीर्णयोः प्रत्ययाविशेषो
भोगः परार्थत्वात्स्वार्थसंयमात्पुरुषज्ञानम्॥३५॥
36. Sattva-puruṣayor atyantāsaṅkīrṇayoḥ praty-
ayāviśeṣo bhogaḥ parārthat svārtha saṁyamāt
puruṣa-jñānam

ततः प्रातिभश्रावणवेदनादर्शास्वादवार्ता
जायन्ते॥३६॥
37. Tataḥ prātibha-śrāvaṇa-vedanādarśāsvā-
da-vārtā jāyante

ते समाधायुपसर्गा व्युत्थाने सद्धियः॥३७॥
38. Te samādhāv upasargā vyutthāne siddhayaḥ

बन्धकारणशैथिल्यात्प्रचारसंवेदनाच्च चित्तस्य
परशरीरावेशः॥३८॥
39. Bandha-kāraṇa-śaithilyāt pracāra-saṁvedanāc
ca cittasya para-śarīrāveśaḥ

उदानजयाज्जलपङ्ककण्टकादिष्विसङ्ग
उत्क्रान्तिश्च॥३९॥
40. Udāna-jayāj jala-paṅka-kaṇṭakādiṣv asaṅga
utkrāntiś ca

*36. Being consciously present in the intellectual mind
and being consciously present in consciousness are two
completely different states of consciousness. By exercising
the samyama on the distinction between the intellect
and Consciousness (purusa), Consciousness can be
experienced.*

*37. This conscious presence in the consciousness gives
the finest hearing, finest feeling, finest sight, finest taste
and finest smell.*

*38. These forces (siddhis) are obstacles to achieving
samādi as they draw attention to the mind.*

*39. When consciousness is unbound and has knowledge
of the flow of energy in the body, it is possible to enter
someone else's body.*

*40. By controlling the life energy (udāna) one can walk
on water, over swamps or thorns, and at will one can
leave the body.*

समानजयाज्ज्वलनम्॥४०॥

41. Samāna-jayāj jvalanam

श्रोत्राकाशयोः सम्बन्धसंयमाद्दवियं श्रोत्रम्॥४१॥

42. Śrotrākāśayoḥ sambandha-saṁyamād divyaṁ
śrotram

कायाकाशयोः सम्बन्धसंयमाल्लघुतूलसमापत्तेश्चाका
शगमनम्॥४२॥

43. Kāyākāśayoḥ sambandha-saṁyamāt lag-
hutūlasamāpatteścakāśagamanam

वहिरकल्पिता वृत्तिर्महाविदिहा ततः
प्रकाशावरणक्षयः॥४३॥

44. Bahir akalpitā vṛttir mahā-videhā tataḥ
prakāśāvaraṇa kṣayaḥ

स्थूलस्वरूपसूक्ष्मान्वयार्थवत्त्वसंयमाद्भूतज
यः॥४४॥

45. Sthūla-svarūpa-sūkṣmānvayārthavattva-saṁy-
amād bhūta-jayaḥ

41. *By controlling the energy samāna (located in the solar plexus), the body can radiate light.*

42. *By exercising the samyama on the connection between hearing and ākāśa (ether or space), divine hearing can be obtained.*

43. *Practicing samyama on the connection between the body and ākāśa results in ease as in cotton fiber, and then the body can fly through the air.*

44. *To consciously free oneself from the limitations of the mind is called mahāvidehā, whereby the veil which hinders the light of distinction can be destroyed.*

45. *By samyama on the qualities of the five elements (bhūtas) as the coarse forms, the subtle constituents and their purpose, the elements can be mastered.*

ततोऽणिमादिप्रादुर्भावः
कायसम्पत्तद्धर्मानभिघातश्च ॥४५॥

46. Tato 'ṇimādi-prādurbhāvaḥ kāya-sampat tad
dharmā anabhighātaś ca

रूपलावण्यबलवज्रसंहननत्वानि कायसम्पत् ॥४६॥

47. Rūpa-lāvaṇya-bala-vajra-saṁhananatvāni
kāya-sampat

ग्रहणस्वरूपास्मितान्वयार्थवत्त्वसंयमादिन्द्रियिज
यः ॥४७॥

48. Grahaṇa-sva-rūpa-āsmitā-anvayārthavatt-
va-saṁyamād indriya-jayaḥ

ततो मनोजवित्वं विकिरणभावः प्रधानजयश्च ॥४८॥

49. Tato manojavitvaṁ vikaraṇa-bhāvaḥ pradhā-
na-jayaś ca

सत्त्वपुरुषान्यताख्यातिमात्रस्य सर्वभावाधिष्ठातृत्वं
सर्वज्ञातृत्वं च ॥४९॥

50. Sattva-puruṣānyatā-khyāti-mātrasya sar-
va-bhāvādhiṣṭhātṛtvaṁ sarvajñātṛtvaṁ ca

46. This gives the ability to change the proportions of the body (animā), such as size. This can lead to the perfection of body and mind.

47. Perfection of the body means beauty, charisma, strength and a firmness like a diamond.

48. Through samyama of the sense organs, their character, quality and purpose as well as the ego (asmitā), a conscious presence arises in the mind and thereby control is gained over it.

49. Through control of the mind, awareness is obtained that is not dependent on body and mind, awareness of the ultimate cause in nature (pradhāna) is established.

50. By performing samyama on the distinction between intellect and consciousness (purusa) omnipotence and omniscience are obtained.

तद्वैराग्यादपि दोषवीजक्षये कैवल्यम्॥५०॥

51. Tad-vairāgyād api doṣa-bīja-kṣaye kaivalyam

स्थान्युपनिमन्त्रणे सङ्गस्मयाकरणं
पुनरनिष्टप्रसङ्गात्॥५१॥

52. Sthāny-upanimantraṇe saṅga smayā-karaṇaṁ
punar aniṣṭa-prasaṅgāt

क्षणतत्क्रमयोः संयमाद्विवेकजं ज्ञानम्॥५२॥

53. Kṣaṇa-tat-kramayoḥ saṁyamād vivekajaṁ
jñānam

जातिलक्षणदेशैरन्यतानवच्छेदात्तुल्ययोस्ततः
परतिपत्तिः॥५३॥

54. Jāti-lakṣaṇa-deśair anyatānavacchedāt tulyay-
os tataḥ pratipattiḥ

तारकं सर्ववषियं सर्वथावषियमक्रमं चेति विवेकजं
ज्ञानम्॥५४॥

55. Tārakaṁ sarva viṣayaṁ sarvathā viṣayam
akramaṁ ceti vivekajaṁ jñānam

सत्त्वपुरुषयोः शुद्धिसाम्ये कैवल्यमिति॥५५॥

56. Sattva-puruṣayoḥ śuddhi sāmye kaivalyam

51. *To renounce these forces means that awareness leaves the seed to the bonds of karma to be liberated and enlightened (kaivalya).*

52. *When heavenly beings are tempting, temptation can lead to false pride and flattery, leading to a fall and to unconsciousness.*

53. *By performing samyamā on the present, knowledge can be obtained through distinction.*

To be consciously present in the now means to be in the now and in eternity at the same time. Being rooted in this level of consciousness means being able to distinguish reality from the illusion, as reality only exists in the present.

54. *By applying this knowledge, two similar objects can be distinguished from each other.*

55. *The highest knowledge arises when there is presence in Consciousness. This knowledge includes everything that can be experienced from the past, in the present, and in the future, and is unbound to time and space.*

56. *Enlightenment (kaivalyam) arises through purification (śuddhi), so that awareness can be present in Consciousness (purusa).*

When mental and physical barriers do not receive atten-tion, awareness can become present in Consciousness.

Chapter 4

KAIVALYA PADA

Enlightenment

जन्मौषधिमन्त्रतपःसमाधिजाः सिद्धयः ॥१॥

1. Janmauṣadhi-mantra-tapaḥ-samādhi-jāḥ siddhayaḥ

जात्यन्तरपरिणामः प्रकृत्यापूरात् ॥२॥

2. Jāty-antara-pariṇāmaḥ prakṛty-āpūrāt

निमित्तमप्रयोजकं प्रकृतीनां वरणभेदस्तु ततः
क्षेत्रिकवत् ॥३॥

3. Nimittam aprayojakaṁ prakṛtīnāṁ varaṇa-bhe-
das tu tataḥ kṣetrikavat

निर्माणचित्तान्यस्मितामात्रात् ॥४॥

4. Nirmāṇa-cittāny asmitā-mātrāt

प्रवृत्तिभेदे प्रयोजकं चित्तमेकमनेकेषाम् ॥५॥

5. Pravṛtti-bhede prayojakaṁ cittam ekam ane-
keṣām

तत्र ध्यानजमनाशयम् ॥६॥

6. Tatra dhyānajam anāśayam

1. The supernatural abilities (siddhis) can be innate or they can arise through drugs (ausadhi), by clean life and abstinence (tapas), by using mantras or being in samādhi.

In Chapter 3, Patanjali describes how siddhis can arise by practicing samyama. They can also occur spontaneously for any of the reasons stated in this sutra.

2. The transition from one level of consciousness to another takes place quite naturally and spontaneously when a level of consciousness has fulfilled its function. In the same way that H2O can change and be liquid water, solid ice or volatile steam, consciousness can change over a period of life.

3. Actions that lead to change are not the cause of the change, they only remove the obstacles to the changes of nature (praktī), such as a farmer who changes the natural flow of water by removing obstacles to the water. At a relative level, there is a constant, ever ongoing change. It is praktī (the relative nature) that is the cause of this constant change. To be only consciously present in this change means to be constantly anchored in the relative. By shifting the focus of attention to the absolute Consciousness, a change can take place. Changing the focus of attention then means a shift from one level of consciousness to another. Actions that remove obstacles can be the practice of pranayama, yoga asanas or meditation which can remove mental imbalance or bodily tensions, which means that the natural flow of life becomes reality in the present.

4. All sensory sensations arise through presence and identification with the ego.

5. All relative mental sensory sensations originate in the nature of the mind (pravritti).

6. Only those mental sensations that arise spontaneously during meditation are free from desire.

कर्माशुक्लाकृष्णं योगिनस्त्रिविधमितरेषाम्॥७॥

7. Karmāśuklākṛṣṇaṁ yoginas tri-vidham itareṣām

ततस्तद्विपाकानुगुणानामेवाभिव्यक्तिर्वासनानाम्॥८॥

8. Tatas tad-vipākānuguṇānām evābhivyaktir
vāsanānām

जातिदेशकालव्यवहितानामप्यानन्तर्यं
स्मृतिसंस्कारयोरेकरूपत्वात्॥९॥

9. Jāti-deśa-kāla-vyavahitānām apy ānantar-yaṁ
smṛti-saṁskārayor ekarūpatvāt

तासामनादित्वं चाशिषो नित्यत्वात्॥१०॥

10. Tāsām anāditvaṁ cāśiṣo nityatvāt

हेतुफलाश्रयालम्बनैः सङ्गृहीतत्वादेषामभावे
तदभावः॥११॥

11. Hetu-phalāśrayālambanaiḥ saṅgṛhītatvād eṣām
abhāve tad-abhāvaḥ

अतीतानागतं स्वरूपतोऽस्त्यध्वभेदाद्धर्माणाम्॥१२॥

12. Atītānāgataṁ svarūpato 'sty adhva-bhedād
dharmāṇām

7. *A yogi's karma is neither dark (unclean) nor light (pure), like the karma of others which is threefold, dark, light or mixed.*

Karma nurtures and teaches through sowing and reaping in the path of life. A yogi who is established and rooted in Consciousness does not need this teaching of life and is therefore independent of karma.

8. *When the circumstances are suitable for threefold karma, karma is manifested, which then bears fruit.*

9. *Through memories and experiences, the cause and effect of karma remain regardless of life situation, time and space.*

10. *The desire to live has always existed and therefore life is eternal.*

It is not always possible to refer to the fact that you have always been alive, this is often because the memory cannot provide information about this. But just because you can not remember and be aware of your first year of life, you do not have to deny that you have been alive this year.

11. *As long as the mind is bound to the cause and effect of karma, awareness is bound to the mind.*

*12. The past and the future exist only as mental sensa-
tions which are distinguished by different characteristics
and qualities.*

ते व्यक्तसूक्ष्मा गुणात्मानः ॥१३॥

13. Te vyakta-sūkṣmā guṇātmānaḥ

परिणामैकत्वाद्वस्तुतत्त्वम् ॥१४॥

14. Pariṇāmaikatvād vastu-tattvam

वस्तुसाम्ये चित्तभेदात्तयोर्विभिक्तः पन्थाः ॥१५॥

15. Vastu-sāmye citta-bhedāt tayor vibhaktaḥ
panthāḥ

न चैकचित्ततन्त्रं वस्तु तदप्रमाणकं तदा किं
स्यात् ॥१६॥

16. Na caika-citta-tantraṁ vastu tad-apramā-ṇa-
kaṁ tadā kiṁ syāt

तदुपरागापेक्षित्वाच्चित्तस्य वस्तु
ज्ञाताज्ञातम् ॥१७॥

17. Tad-uparāgāpekṣitvāc cittasya vastu
jñātājñātam

सदा ज्ञाताश्चित्तवृत्तयस्तत्प्रभोः
पुरुषस्यापरिणामित्वात् ॥१८॥

18. Sadā jñātāś citta-vṛttayas tat-prabhoḥ
puruṣasyāpariṇāmitvāt

13. They can be manifest or unmanifest and have different characteristics and qualities (gunās).

14. The unique state of an object in the present depends
on the influence of the three gunās and this applies to all
relative existence.

15. Sensory perceptions are experienced differently depending on the level of consciousness that prevails.

16. An object is not dependent on a single mind, if so,
what would happen if an object is not experienced by
this mind?

Although the sensory perceptions of an object are mental experiences, an object has its own existence whether
it is experienced or not.

17. An object can only be experienced if the sense per-
ception is present for consciousness.

If consciousness is rooted in thoughts other than what
is happening in the present, the experience of an object
can be lost.

18. All changes in the mind are witnessed by Consciousness which is constantly the unchanging observer.

न तत्स्वाभासं दृश्यत्वात्॥१९॥

19. Na tat svābhāsaṁ dṛśyatvāt

एकसमये चोभयानवधारणम्॥२०॥

20. Eka-samaye cobhayānavadhāraṇam

चित्तान्तरदृश्ये बुद्धिबुद्धेरतिप्रसङ्गः
स्मृतिसङ्करश्च॥२१॥

21. Cittāntara-dṛśye buddhi-buddher ati-pra-
saṅgaḥ smṛti-saṅkaraś ca

चितिरप्रतिसङ्क्रमायास्तदाकारापत्तौ
स्वबुद्धिसंवेदनम्॥२२॥

22. Citerapratisaṅkramāyāstadākārāpattau sva-
buddhisaṁvedanam

द्रष्टृदृश्योपरक्तं चित्तं सर्वार्थम्॥२३॥

23. Draṣṭṛdṛśyoparaktaṁ cittaṁ sarvārtham

19. The mind is not self-enlightened, although it is perceptible.

Like the moon which does not shine by itself but by the rays of the sun, the mind is illuminated only by Consciousness. The mind is a tool for sensory sensations to become aware.

20. Since the mind is not self-enlightened, it cannot be consciously present in both the senses and in Consciousness at the same time.

Being anchored in the mind and consciously present in the sensory sensations does not mean simultaneous presence in Consciousness. Only by being consciously anchored in the Consciousness can conscious presence arise in both the mind and Consciousness at the same time.

21. If the mind could be experienced by another mind, confusion would arise as to which mind belongs to memories and sensory perceptions.

At the level of relative existence, it is necessary that each mind is delimited and limited to an individual consciousness, so that the life situation does not become chaotic and incomprehensible.

22. Consciousness is immutable, but when awareness identifies with the changing intellect (buddhi) and the senses of the mind it loses contact with Consciousness.

23. Awareness is colored by both the observing absolute Consciousness and the observed relative objects.

तदसङ्ख्येयवासनाभिश्चित्रमपि परार्थं
संहत्यकारित्वात् ॥२४॥

24. Tadasaṅkhyeyavāsanābhiścitramapi parārtham
saṁhatyakāritvāt

विशेषदर्शिन आत्मभावभावनाविनिवृत्तिः॥२५॥
25. Viśeṣa-darśina ātma-bhāva-bhāvanā-vinivṛttiḥ

तदा विवेकनिम्नङ्कैवल्यप्राग्भारञ्चित्तम्॥२६॥
26. Tadā viveka-nimnaṁ kaivalya-prāg-bhāraṁ
cittam

तच्छिद्रेषु प्रत्ययान्तराणि संस्कारेभ्यः॥२७॥
27. Tac chidreṣu pratyayāntarāṇi saṁskārebhyaḥ

हानमेषां क्लेशवदुक्तम्॥२८॥
28. Hānameṣāṁ kleśavad uktam

प्रसङ्ख्यानेऽप्यकुसीदस्य सर्वथा
विविकख्यातेर्धर्ममेघः समाधिः॥२९॥
29. Prasaṅkhyāne 'py akusīdasya sarvathā vive-
ka-khyāter dharma-meghaḥ samādhiḥ

24. Awareness affected by various senses and desires
(vāsanās) is dependent on Consciousness and its higher
purpose.

25. He who is consciously present in Consciousness
ceases to seek his identity in sensory perceptions in the
mind and ego.

26. Then, when awareness has the ability to distinguish
and observe (viveka) the sensory sensations (cittam),
absolute freedom (kaivalya) can arise.

27. When awareness does not have the ability to distinguish and observe thoughts and feelings from past,
experiences will affect awareness.

There is an individual bank of experiences that lies latent and is activated by memory and becomes conscious
with the help of thoughts and feelings. If awareness is
not consciously present and can observe and distinguish
in the present, the past experiences will automatically
be activated to help with appropriate information from
the past.

28. These can be removed in the same way as other
disorders that lead to suffering (kleśas).

Some thoughts and feelings from past experiences can be an obstacle to presence in Consciousness and the state of yoga. Therefore, their influence over awareness must be overcome and removed.

29. Then this constant, selfless, distinctive, state of consciousness has resulted in the ultimate supreme state where awareness "from a cloud giving rain in the form of heavenly virtue and grace "dharma meghah samādhih".

When awareness is present in consciousness, this state gives total satisfaction and then there is no need to seek more satisfaction. That the mind should try to intellectually suffocate obstacles that arise in the form of thoughts and feelings is ineffective when they are back sooner or later. That is, awareness as through "a rain in the form of heavenly virtue and grace" (dharma meghah samādhih) that can do this and bring awareness in Consciousness. The mind can be helpful to the awareness by being cooperative and e.g. apply one or more of the eightfold paths; yama, niyama, asanas, pranayama, pratyahara, dharana, dhyana and samadhi, but it is the grace of God that ultimately establishes the consciousness of Samadhi.

तत: क्लेशकर्मनिवृत्ति:॥३०॥

30. Tataḥ kleśa-karma-nivṛttiḥ

तदा सर्वावरणमलापेतस्य ज्ञानस्यानन्त्याज्ज्ञेयम
ल्पम्॥३१॥

31. Tadā sarvāvaraṇa-malāpetasya jñānasyā-nan-
tyāj jñeyam alpam

तत: कृतार्थानां परिणामक्रमसमाप्तिर्गुणानाम्॥३२॥

32. Tataḥ kṛtārthānāṁ pariṇāma-krama-samāptir
guṇānām

क्षणप्रतियोगी परिणामापरान्तनिर्ग्राह्य:
क्रम:॥३३॥

33. Kṣaṇa-pratiyogī pariṇāmāparānta-nirgrāhyaḥ
kramaḥ

पुरुषार्थशून्यानां गुणानां प्रतिप्रसव: कैवल्यं
स्वरूपप्रतिष्ठा वा चितिशक्तिरिति॥३४॥

34. Puruṣārtha-śūnyānāṁ guṇānāṁ pratiprasavaḥ
kaivalyaṁ svarūpa-pratiṣṭhā vā citi-śakter iti

30. Then all disturbances and obstacles cease, as well as the effects of karma that cause suffering.

31. When distractions and obstacles have been removed, knowledge emerges that cannot be compared with the limited intellectual knowledge of the mind.

Different types of disturbances and obstacles from the experience bank then no longer fill any function. Of course, useful experiences from the past can be used in the present.

32. Once the state of dharma meghah samādhi is established, the three gunas (tamas, rajas and sattva) have fulfilled their duties.

The three gunas have tasks to perform and when that is done, they have finished playing their roles in the arena of the mind.

33. Kramah is an element of the constant change that takes place in the eternal present and can be experienced when the three gunas are transformed.

In parallel with the constant change in the relative existence, there is the absolute eternal immutable being. The changing existence can only be experienced by its opposite, the unchanging being.

34. Kaivalya is the state of consciousness that arises
when the three gunas no longer affect, as they no longer
have any purpose to fill. Then awareness is present in
the real state of consciousness which is pure Consciousness.

Postscript

Patanjalis Yoga Sutras can be seen as a handbook in describing the real and the illusory existence. Ie., to be present in the eternal absolute pure Consciousness and to be bound by the perishable relative existence. Patanjali's sutras are characterized by nondualism, ie., that there is no contradiction between the absolute Consciousness and the relative mind and ego. There is only one Consciousness at the absolute level, only the degree of awareness is different at the relative level.

The basic purpose is not to create a belief system with intellectual interpretations but to provide an accurate description of the yogic process that can be verified through one's own experiences of Yoga and the state of consciousness Samadhi. It is possible to look at the sutras from a scientific philosophical perspective. It then becomes a dualistic view whose purpose is to do scientific research, investigate and compare the sutras, not to transcend the mind to be present in Yoga, Samadhi.

Ultimately, it is the Yoga and state of consciousness, Samadhi that provides confirmation and contributes to an identity shift from bondage in mind to presence in Consciousness . The change of identity takes place when there is sufficient maturity for it. This does not mean that the intellect and senses disappear but that they are refined.

With Ashtanga Yoga, Patanjali describes eight different tools to help establish awareness in Consciousness that is constantly present and eternal. The purpose of the sutras and the aids he proposes is that constant presence in Consciousness, in Yoga, shall be established.

By applying samyama to Patanjali's sutras, qualities such as kindness, compassion, humility, and selflessness can be established and inner peace, happiness, and harmony can arise in life.

Tat Tvam Asi - Thou art That.

Om shanti shanti shanti!